I Care

Words of Encouragement for Caregivers

Wendy Albouy

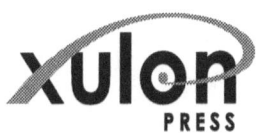

Copyright © 2006 by Wendy Albouy

I Care
by Wendy Albouy

Printed in the United States of America

ISBN 1-60034-012-1

All rights reserved solely by the author. The author guarantees all contents are original and do not infringe upon the legal rights of any other person or work. No part of this book may be reproduced in any form without the permission of the author. The views expressed in this book are not necessarily those of the publisher.

Unless otherwise indicated, Bible quotations are taken from the King James Version of the Bible Copyright © 1994 by The Zondervan Corporation.

www.xulonpress.com

In loving memory of

Carol Ann Albouy
My mother

and

Catherine Almira Trott Hodgson
My grandmother

Table of Contents

Introduction ix

As a caregiver I feel
weak in mind, body, and spirit 11

As a caregiver I feel angry 15

As a caregiver I feel lonely 21

As a caregiver I dread the
Christmas holidays 25

As a caregiver I feel afraid 31

As a caregiver I feel helpless 37

As a caregiver I can't believe
how insensitive people can be 41

As a caregiver I feel discouraged 47

Reflections 53

A Caregiver's Prayer 55

Introduction

*I*f you are taking care of a sick loved one or if you know someone else who is, you realize how much of a twenty-four-hour job this can be. Life is no longer as it used to be, and sometimes dealing with the many emotions that accompany caregiving can be difficult.

My mother was fifty-two years old when she was diagnosed with breast cancer, and as her illness progressed my family shared in her caregiving. This experience allowed my siblings and me the opportunity to bond with our mother in ways that would not have been possible if she had never gotten sick.

We knew our mother felt safe and loved, and she appreciated all we did for her. We are secure in the knowledge that we did all we could to make a difference in the comfort of our mother's life, and we will treasure these memories forever. We acknowledge that we could not have made it this far without God on our side, because without Him we would have been lost.

Sadly, on Mother's Day 2002 our mother passed away after battling cancer for three years. She remained faithful to God during the entire ordeal, and her life was a testimony of His goodness and mercy. Although her passing was a tremendous loss for us, we are hopeful because we know that in her death our prayers for her healing were answered. We believe she is now completely healed and her spirit dwells in perfect peace with God.

Today I am a more caring person who is sensitive to the needs of those who are sick. I am fully in touch with the human experience of pain and suffering because I have lived it firsthand. My heart goes out to caregivers all over the world who fulfill a role that can be draining and rewarding simultaneously.

It is my sincere prayer that this book touch the lives of other caregivers who may feel they are all alone. I pray this message helps others to realize there are countless people out there who are experiencing the same things daily.

Although my entire family helped to care for my mother, this book is my own account of caregiving and the direct impact it had on my life.

Wendy Albouy

*As a caregiver
I feel weak in mind, body,
and spirit*

Some days it was very difficult for me to visit my mother when she was hospitalized. I dreaded walking the long and lonely corridor that led to the hospital elevators.

Daily I would spend my lunch hours and evenings at her bedside, and after a while I found myself becoming drained physically, emotionally, and spiritually.

How God helped me to become a stronger person:

When I realized that the God of Comfort understood how I felt even if no one else did, His strength allowed me to have the mental, physical, and spiritual strength I needed day after day as I visited my mother. By His grace and mercy I was able to endure the rigors of caregiving.

A caregiver's prayer for strength:

Dear God,

Grant me the strength I need to endure another day. Some days I feel so exhausted as I try to juggle my daily routines and care for my loved one. Help me to stay well so I can take care of my loved one. Give me the peace I need to get a good night's sleep, eat properly, and care for myself as well. All these things I ask in Jesus' name. Amen.

Matthew 11:28
> Come unto me, all ye that labour and are heavy laden, and I will give you rest.

*As a caregiver
I feel angry*

I admit I wrestled with feelings of anger and resentment when my mother got sick. I know she didn't ask to be ill, and I wasn't actually angry at her. I was mad at the situation and the circumstances. Life seemed so unfair. She was young and vibrant, and I was angry at all we had to endure.

Sometimes it felt as though everyone around me was living happy and stress-free lives while I was constantly trying to cope.

When she became critically ill I got angry with the hospital staff, who tried to explain her condition was deteriorating.

How God helped me to deal with my anger:

Becoming angry at what appeared to be an unfair situation was normal, but when I realized God was in control of everything that happened and I was not alone in it, my feelings of anger began to subside.

My mother got the best medical care possible, and I understood that the doctors and administrators were only trying their best to handle a very delicate situation. I have learned to channel those feelings of anger into a positive direction that allows me to reach out and help others who are going through a similar situation.

A caregiver's prayer for overcoming anger:

Dear God,

You know how angry I feel when I think of how carefree life used to be and how much things have changed since my loved one got ill. Help me not to resent the happiness others around me experience. Help me to realize that doctors and other hospital staff are there to provide the best care for my loved one. Show me how to channel my feelings of anger positively so You can receive all the glory and honor You deserve.

All these things I ask in Jesus' name. Amen.

Ephesians 4:26
   Be ye angry, and sin not: let not the sun go down upon your wrath.

As a caregiver
I feel lonely

It was difficult for me to observe other mothers and daughters together. I was very close with my mother, and during her illness I longed for the days when we used to travel together. Her weakness did not allow her to do the things she used to do, and I grieved for this part of our relationship before she even passed away.

Those who still have their mothers have no idea how blessed they are, and it upsets me when I observe someone taking their mother for granted.

How God helped me to deal with my feelings of loneliness:

Feelings of loneliness are very real, and it took me a long time to deal with the shock of not having around the mother I remembered from my childhood. God showed me that the years I did get to spend with my mother were a blessing.

Many others have never known their mothers for various reasons, and the memories I have of happy times spent together will remain in my heart forever. I am now able to encourage others not to take for granted the fact that their mothers are alive and well.

A caregiver's prayer for overcoming loneliness:

Dear God,

You know how much I ache to have my loved one active and well again. I miss all the times we spent together doing activities such as traveling and playing sports. Even the everyday tasks such as grocery shopping, cooking, or watching TV together are no longer possible because the illness has made my loved one's body weak.

Lord, I pray for Your presence each day. Help me to also value the lives of those around me who are well, and let me not take for granted their presence in my life. All these things I ask in Jesus' name. Amen.

Hebrews 13:5
    I will never leave thee, nor forsake thee.

*As a caregiver
I dread the Christmas
holidays*

Holidays can be difficult when you are caring for a loved one. My mother's very last Christmas was bittersweet. She had just come home from receiving eight weeks of radiation treatment, and she was very weak. The whole family was excited at her homecoming, and we decorated the house with Christmas decorations much earlier than we normally would have just to surprise her. When she arrived home and saw how beautiful things were she was elated. I will never forget how happy she was.

Since early childhood Christmas has always been very special to me. This time of year is definitely a challenge now because I no longer have my mother. Sounds of familiar Christmas music always take me back to a time when things were so different. It is amazing how memories of childhood remain with us no matter how old we are. Whenever I hear the first sounds of beloved Christmas carols I feel sentimental.

How God helped me to face Christmas:

The true meaning of Christmas is the birth of Jesus Christ. He came to this earth to save each and every person from sin. God has shown me that Christmas is not a time for me to dread but a time to remember the love He showed to mankind. This act of love is an example of how I can reach out to help others who may also be having a difficult time during the holidays.

Sometimes if I am caught off guard by a Christmas carol I allow myself to cry because it is cleansing to my soul and essential to my healing. I relish the memories of past Christmases while I also try to create new memories with family and friends I am still blessed to have in my life.

A caregiver's prayer for facing Christmas:

Dear God,

Winter is approaching and pretty soon the familiar sounds of carols and bustling shoppers will become a part of my daily life. While I am caring for my loved one it is difficult to be happy about this time of the year. Help me to understand that it is okay to feel sad. Help me not to put too much pressure on myself to have a picture-perfect Christmas gathering like those shown on television. Life is not perfect, and even if I am not able to buy gifts and cook a turkey, I am thankful for all that You have done for me this year. Thank You for another opportunity to show others the kind of love You showed the world when You gave Your Son as a gift to this earth.

All these things I ask in Jesus' name. Amen.

John 3:16
>For God so loved the world, that He gave His only begotten son.

*As a caregiver
I feel afraid*

It frightened me to see how much the treatments and cancer altered my mother's appearance. She was always beautiful, even up to the day she died, but her petite body was so thin and frail.

For the first two years of her illness no one could look at her and detect that she was sick. However, when she began her radiation treatments I was shocked to see how damaging it was to her skin. I would help her to bathe each night, and the first time I saw the burns on her back from the treatment I was very afraid. No one explained to me that this would happen, and even if they had I believe I would have reacted the same way.

I tried to act normal as I washed her back, and I don't think she fully realized how much damage was done to her skin. I was thankful she wasn't able to see her back. It sickened me to see her body undergo so much abuse in the way of needles, medication, and burns.

How God helped me to deal with the toll the illness took on my mother's body:

Once the cancer began to take a physical toll on my mother's body it was hard to accept, but God showed me that no matter what suffering she had to go through He would never leave us. While she received her radiation I had the opportunity to sit in a small waiting room with many other caregivers who were waiting for their loved ones. We all shared a common bond, and although it was difficult to watch each person as they entered the waiting area, I had comfort in knowing we were not alone in our suffering, and that there were many other families out there who also were undergoing cancer treatments.

A caregiver's prayer for help to deal with overcoming fear:

Dear God,

You know how much it breaks my heart to see the physical and emotional changes that my loved one has gone through. I miss the familiar appearance I used to know.

When I enter my loved one's hospital room, help me to be mindful of the fact that there are no mirrors around, and my loved one, who knows me so very well, will read my facial expressions. Lord, help my face not to express shock and dismay as I behold the physical changes that have taken place. Help me to be more like You who sees the beauty on the inside of a person. Help me to tell them how good they look because You know the healing power of words spoken in loving kindness.

All these things I ask in Jesus' name. Amen.

2 Timothy 1:7
    For God hath not given us the spirit of fear; but of power, and of love, and of a sound mind.

*As a caregiver
I feel helpless*

Sometimes I became frustrated because I felt helpless. I always wanted to make the situation better for my mother, but I didn't know how.

As her caregiver I sometimes felt that I was not doing enough. She never made me feel this way, but I put that pressure on myself.

How God helped me not to feel helpless:

God showed me that the little things in life do make a big difference. He was able to provide my mother with everything she needed. He gave me wisdom to discern when she needed a boost to her spirit. There came a time when I realized that all the money in the world would not make her life better, but something as small as bringing a gospel tape for her to listen to in the hospital really made her happy and helped her to sleep at night. When she was at home and in a lot of pain I held a washcloth on her forehead and sat up with her sometimes until 2:00 a.m. just so she wouldn't feel alone. Even something as simple as giving her a pen to write with while she was in the hospital, combing her hair, or giving her a bath was enough to make her feel good. I believe God directed my every gesture and allowed me to anticipate her basic needs.

A caregiver's prayer for help to deal with feelings of helplessness:

Dear God,

Help me to be mindful of the little things in life that could make my loved one more comfortable. Show me the needs that my loved one might not even be able to express to me. You are all knowing and able to impress upon my heart exactly what to do. Help me to depend on You at all times because only You know everything it will take to care for my loved one.

All these things I ask in Jesus' name. Amen.

Philippians 4:19
> But my God shall supply all your need according to His riches in glory by Christ Jesus.

*As a caregiver
I can't believe how
insensitive people can be*

*G*enerally speaking most people are kind and compassionate when dealing with the sick and their families, but there were times when my mother and I encountered insensitive people.

One particular day when she was in the hospital I stopped by to visit and she was very upset. Apparently a stranger had entered her room to visit one of the other patients in her room. This person began to gossip loudly about the poor health condition of someone who was dying of cancer. This is the type of person that no hospital room needs.

I also recalled my mother telling me there were times when she was lying in her bed with her eyes closed and visitors would come and stand over her and talk negatively about her appearance. These unknowing visitors thought she wasn't listening, but she heard every word loud and clear.

People need to be mindful of what they say in the presence of a sick person. Negative comments can damage the spirit of someone who is already in a fragile condition.

How God helped me to deal with insensitive people:

I Care

My natural reaction was disbelief that there were actually people who talked negatively over a sick person. God showed me that these people are insensitive because they have not experienced what it is like to care for a loved one. He showed me that that is exactly the type of person I should strive not to be like. I had to show compassion for people who lacked sensitivity because they truly didn't know any better. I now know how to inspire others when I visit them in the hospital or at home, and I know how not to bring down their spirits.

A caregiver's prayer for help in dealing with insensitive people:

Dear God,

Help me not to be the type of person who is insensitive to others. Help me to monitor who comes in contact with my sick loved one so that I may protect them from anyone who enters the sick room with a negative spirit. Help me to also remember that a sleeping sick person is still able to hear words that are spoken over them.

Give me the words to comfort my loved one if an insensitive comment is made. Help me to have tolerance toward those who are unable to use discretion in these situations.

All these things I ask in Jesus' name. Amen.

Psalm 23:4
   …thy rod and thy staff they comfort me.

*As a caregiver
I feel discouraged*

I felt very discouraged when my mother's health really became poor. She spent the last three weeks of her life in the hospital. Everything felt like it was happening in slow motion. I had been so hopeful that she would overcome the disease, especially after she was told she was cancer free following her treatments.

My relief turned to dismay when four months after she was told she was cancer free she became incredibly weak. Her decline was rapid, and once she was admitted to the hospital there was one bad report after another.

The cancer had spread to her bones and her brain. I stood there in disbelief as the doctor relayed her test results.

How God helped me deal with my feelings of discouragement.

This was really the lowest point of her entire illness, but God is good because He was able to give me hope even in my mother's very last hours on this earth.

I was in her room the day before she died, and I had a little radio playing gospel music. By this time she was on such heavy painkillers I was no longer able to have a conversation with her. I tried to communicate but she would only give me a glassy stare that looked almost through me. As the radio played a familiar song my mother suddenly began to sing the song loud and clear. I was so shocked; I had no idea she even noticed the radio playing. God is really good because He showed me mercy and kindness even in my darkest hour. This is a memory that gives me hope because I know that no matter what the doctor said about her, only God had the final say in the matter and He took her home when all her work on this earth was completed.

I was meant to hear her angelic voice sing one last time. For a brief moment it felt like things were back to normal. Although she never again got to come back to her home on earth, I know without a doubt that she went home to be with the Lord who watched over her every step of the way through her illness.

A caregiver's prayer for help in dealing with feelings of discouragement:

Dear God,

Even in my darkest hours help me to realize that You are the God of hope who controls all things. Even when the doctors deliver bad news, help me to remember that only You have the final say in all things.

Have mercy on me and give me hope even when everything around me seems so hopeless.

All these things I ask in Jesus' name. Amen.

1 Peter 5:7
   Casting all your care upon Him: for He careth for you.

Reflections

A caregiver gives love, time, attention, meals, baths, companionship, and so much more.

God is the ultimate caregiver who loves and cares for each one of His children.

Let His love wash over you as you bathe your loved one.

Feed your mind, body, and soul with His Word as you provide, cook, and serve meals for your loved one.

While you comb your loved one's hair remember God knows the number of hairs on your head, and that is how well He cares about you and your well being.

When you sit beside the sickbed and hold your loved one's hand, remember God sits beside you and is there to hold your hand as well.

As you care for your sick loved one remember God loved you first and He can help you get through the many emotions you will experience as you administer care to the one you love so dearly.

Be encouraged and be blessed.

A Caregiver's Prayer

Dear Lord,

Surround me with Your presence,
as I care throughout my day.

Hold my hand and guide me,
in Your warm and loving way.

Calm my many fears
with Your tender love.

Strength and patience for today,
are blessings from above.

When I feel alone,
remind me that You're there.

Bonding with my loved one,
is a gift revealed through care.

Wendy Albouy

To contact Wendy please email:

wendy_albouy5@hotmail.com

www.ingramcontent.com/pod-product-compliance
Lightning Source LLC
Chambersburg PA
CBHW021038180526
45163CB00005B/2185